AF392362

Table of Contents

When shopping at the grocery store, the foods you grab can greatly impact your overall health. In fact, filling your cart with a lot of refined grains, sugary drinks, and processed foods can increase inflammation and affect your health.

Therefore, filling up on healthy foods can help keep you healthy, protect against chronic diseases resistant to drugs and rid your body of toxins.

We also absorb tons of toxins every day through the air we breathe, the water we drink, the food we eat, and by just being outside in our surroundings.

So how do we get rid of these toxins that can be harmful to our body? It's through the Healing diet.

The Healing foods diet is not just a diet; It is a tool that will lead you to a total transformation of your health. This diet was designed to help everyone overcome diseases. It is designed to heal your body and improve your health by encouraging the consumption of nutritious, whole foods like fruits, veggies, legumes, healthy fats, organic meats, and healing herbs and spices.

Plus, this simple eating pattern is a great way to ensure you supply your body with a steady stream of the nutrients you need to help prevent nutritional deficiencies in your diet and to promote healthy living.

So what makes this diet unique?

This diet is unique because it involves making some simple switches in your diet compared to other complicated diets with many rules and regulations.

1. Maple BBQ Salmon with Brown Butter Couscous

Prep: 15 mins

Cook: 30 mins

Total: 45 mins

Servings: 4

Ingredients

- 2 pounds salmon filets
- 1 tablespoon brown sugar
- 1 teaspoon garlic powder
- 1 teaspoon smoked paprika
- ½ teaspoon salt
- ½ teaspoon freshly ground black pepper
- ¼ teaspoon cumin
- 2 to 3 tablespoons maple syrup

Brown Butter Couscous

- 1 tablespoon unsalted butter

- 1 cup uncooked pearl couscous

- 1 ¼ cups chicken or vegetable stock

- A pinch of salt

- 2 tablespoons unsalted butter

- 1 garlic clove, minced

Directions

1. Preheat the oven to 400 degrees F. Place the salmon on a baking sheet.

2. In a small bowl, whisk together the sugar, garlic powder, paprika, salt, pepper and cumin. Sprinkle it all over the salmon filets. Drizzle each filet with the maple syrup and use a spoon to spread it all over the filet.

3. Roast for 10 to 15 minutes, until the salmon just flakes with a fork. If desired, you can brush with a little more maple syrup when it comes out of the oven. Top with chopped chives. Serve immediately with brown butter couscous.

Brown butter couscous

1. Heat a large saucepan over medium heat and add the butter. Stir in the couscous until coated, then cook for 2 to 3 minutes, stirring, until the couscous is slightly toasty. Add in the stock and salt and bring the mixture to a boil. Once boiling, reduce to a simmer and cover. Cook for 15 minutes, or until the liquid is absorbed.

2. While the couscous is cooking, heat a small saucepan over medium heat and add the butter. Cook, whisking often, until brown bits appear on the bottom of the pan. Remove the butter from the heat and stir in the garlic cloves.

3. Once the couscous is finished, drizzle with the garlic brown butter. Toss and serve.

2. Teriyaki Shrimp Sushi Bowl

Prep: 5 mins

Cook: 15 mins

Total: 20 mins

Servings: 2

Ingredients

- 1 cup cooked white rice
- ½ cup cooked quinoa
- 1 teaspoon olive oil
- ½ lb. cooked shrimp, thawed
- 3 garlic cloves minced
- ¼ cup teriyaki sauce
- 1 tablespoon sesame seeds
- ¾ cup cucumber sliced
- 1 avocado sliced

For the teriyaki sauce:

- ¼ cup soy sauce
- 2 tablespoon maple syrup

- 1 tablespoon rice vinegar

- ½ teaspoon fresh ginger, grated

- 1 tablespoon cornstarch

For the spicy mayo:

- 2 tablespoon mayonnaise

- 1 teaspoon sriracha or more to taste

Directions

1. If you haven't already, cook the rice and quinoa then set them aside, keeping a lid on the saucepan(s) so they stay warm.

2. Add oil and shrimp to a large skillet, then sauté the shrimp over medium heat for 2-3 minutes. While the shrimp is heating up, make the teriyaki sauce by whisking all of the sauce ingredients together.

3. Next, add the garlic to the skillet and sauté for 1 minute. Reduce the heat to low, then pour ¼ cup of the teriyaki sauce into the pan, using a wooden spoon to stir until the shrimp is coated. Remove

from the heat, then sprinkle the shrimp with sesame seeds.

4. Assemble: Add the rice/quinoa mixture to a bowl, then top it with the marinated shrimp, cucumber and avocado. Drizzle the remaining teriyaki sauce over top.

5. Last, whisk the mayo and sriracha together, then drizzle that over top of everything.

3. Apricot Chicken Thighs with Root Vegetables

Prep: 15 mins

Cook: 17 mins

Total: 32 mins

Servings: 4

Ingredients

- 1 tablespoon olive oil
- 20 ounces Organic Boneless Skinless Chicken Thighs
- Kosher salt and fresh ground black pepper to taste
- 2/3 cup low sodium chicken broth
- 1/4 cup apricot preserves
- 2 tablespoons Dijon mustard
- 1 cup diced carrots
- 1 cup diced parsnips
- 1 cup diced rutabaga
- 1 teaspoon finely chopped fresh sage
- 1 teaspoon finely chopped fresh rosemary

- 1 teaspoon finely chopped fresh thyme

- 1 1/2 teaspoons grated garlic (2-3 cloves)

Directions

1. Heat the olive oil in a large skillet over medium-high heat. Season the chicken thighs with salt and pepper then add them to the hot skillet. Cook approximately 3-4 minutes per side or until golden brown. The chicken won't be fully cooked at this point. Remove the chicken from the skillet and onto a plate.

2. Whisk together the chicken broth, apricot preserves and Dijon in a small bowl and set aside.

3. Add the carrots, parsnips and rutabaga to the skillet, season with salt and pepper and sauté 4-5 minutes. Add in the herbs and garlic and sauté another minute.

4. Add the chicken back into the skillet and pour in the apricot mixture. Reduce the heat to medium, cover with a lid or piece of foil and cook for

another 7-8 minutes or until the chicken is cooked through.

5. Once the chicken is cooked, taste for seasoning and spoon some of the sauce over the chicken thighs. Garnish with more fresh herbs then serve.

4. Teriyaki Ground Turkey Skillet with Vegetables

Prep: 15 mins

Cook: 30 mins

Total: 45 mins

Servings: 4

Ingredients

- 2 tbsp avocado oil
- 1/2 red onion, finely chopped
- 2 large carrots, peeled and chopped
- 1 bunch radishes, chopped
- 1 tbsp fresh ginger, peeled and grated
- 1 pound ground turkey
- 1/4 cup teriyaki sauce
- 2 medium zucchini squash, chopped
- 2 cups baby spinach,
- 1/2 tsp sea salt, to taste

For Serving (Optional)

- 1 bunch chives, chopped

- 1 tbsp sesame seeds

Directions

1. Heat the oil in a large (12-inch) skillet with deep sides over medium heat. Add the red onion and cook, stirring occasionally, until onion begins to soften, about 3 minutes. Add the carrots, radishes, and ginger. Cover and cook 3 minutes.

2. Scoot the vegetables off to one side of the skillet and add the ground turkey. Brown on one side for 2 to 3 minutes, then flip and continue browning another 2 minutes. Give everything a big stir to combine it all together.

3. Add the teriyaki sauce, chopped zucchini, spinach, and sea salt. Cover and cook until turkey has cooked through and vegetables have reached desired done-ness, about 4 to 5 minutes.

4. Serve with chopped chives and sesame seeds.

5. Banh mi bowls with sticky tofu

Prep: 15 mins

Cook: 15 mins

Total: 30 mins

Servings: 2

Ingredients

Sticky tofu:

- 1 pack tofu
- 2 tbsp avocado oil (or other high heating oil)
- 1 tbsp soy sauce (regular or gluten-free)
- 2 tbsp hoisin sauce (regular or gluten-free)
- 1 tsp Sriracha

Bowls:

- 1/2 pack rice noodles
- 1 cup shredded lettuce
- 1/2 cup thinly sliced or shredded carrots
- 1/2 cup thinly sliced cucumbers

- 1/2 cup shredded red cabbage, or picked red cabbage
- 1 handful cilantro, chopped
- 1 avocado, sliced
- sesame seeds for topping

Directions

1. Chop the tofu into cubes, and place in a hot pan with the oil on medium-high heat.
2. Allow to brown, approximately 3-5 minutes, and then flip the cubes to brown on each side.
3. Once each side is golden brown and crispy, turn off the heat, and toss the soy sauce, hoisin sauce, and Sriracha.
4. Cook the rice noodles according to the package directions.
5. Place your bowl with the noodles on the bottom, and top tofu, lettuce, carrots, cucumber, red cabbage, cilantro, avocado, and sesame seeds.
6. Top with extra soy sauce and hoisin sauce.

Prep: 5 mins

Cook: 20 mins

Total: 25 mins

Servings: 4

Ingredients

For the Sauce:

- 6 tbsp low sodium-soy sauce
- 1 tbsp hoisin sauce
- 3/4 tbsp apple cider vinegar
- 2 tbsp honey
- 1 tsp toasted sesame oil
- 1/2 tsp fresh minced ginger
- 2 cloves garlic minced
- 2 tbsp cornstarch
- 1/2 cup water plus more as needed to thin out sauce

For the chicken and vegetables:

- 2 medium skinless boneless chicken thighs or breasts cut into 1" inch cubes
- Salt and black pepper to taste
- 1 1/2 cups broccoli florets about 1 head
- 1 red bell pepper cut into chunks
- 1/2 green bell pepper cut into chunks (optional - for extra color)
- 2/3 cup roasted unsalted cashews

Optional garnishes

- Toasted sesame seeds and chopped green onions

Directions

For the sauce:

1. In a medium saucepan over medium heat, whisk together soy sauce, hoisin sauce, vinegar, honey, sesame oil, garlic, ginger, cornstarch and water until combined. Bring to a simmer, stirring frequently, until sauce thickens and bubbles. Remove from heat and set aside.

For the chicken and vegetables

1. Preheat oven to 400°, line a large sheet pan with parchment paper or foil coated with cooking spray and set aside.

2. Season chicken with salt and black pepper then drizzle spoonfuls of sauce over the chicken coating well on both sides. Reserve at least half of the sauce for later.

3. Cook in preheated oven for 8 minutes then remove the pan.

4. Arrange the broccoli florets, bell peppers and cashews in a single layer around the chicken. Season the vegetables with salt and pepper and drizzle spoonfuls of the sauce and toss everything to coat. Return to the oven and cook for another 8-12 minutes, or until the chicken is cooked through and juices run clear.

5. Remove pan from oven and drizzle with remaining sauce. Serve over rice or quinoa and garnish with green onions and sesame seeds, if desired.

7. Roasted Vegetable Lasagna

Prep: 45 mins

Cook: 50 mins

Total: 1 hr 35 mins

Servings: 8

Ingredients

- 12-15 lasagna noodles
- Roasted Vegetables
- 2 large broccoli crowns, broken into florets
- 8 oz. sliced mushrooms
- 1 red bell pepper, chopped
- 1 onion, chopped
- 1 zucchini, chopped
- Olive oil
- Salt
- Pepper
- Bechamel Sauce
- 5 tbsp. butter

- ¼ cup flour

- 4 cups milk

- 2 tsp. salt

- ¼ tsp. nutmeg

- 2 tbsp. fresh herbs

- ½ tsp. garlic powder

Cheese:

- 24 oz. cottage cheese or ricotta cheese

- ½ cup finely grated Parmesan cheese

- ½ tsp. salt

- ¼ tsp. ground black pepper

- ½ tsp. garlic powder

- 1 tsp. dried oregano

- 1 tsp. dried basil

- 16 oz. shredded mozzarella cheese

Directions

1. Bring a large pot of salted water to a boil and prepare lasagna noodles according to package

directions. Drain and set aside. Drizzle with olive oil to prevent sticking.

2. Preheat oven to 400 degrees Fahrenheit. Spread vegetables over two sheet pans and drizzle with olive oil. Sprinkle with salt and pepper and use your hands to toss to coat. Bake for 25-30 minutes until tender and remove from oven to cool.

3. Meanwhile, make your béchamel sauce. Melt butter in a large saucepan. Whisk in flour and stir until full incorporated. Whisk in milk, salt, nutmeg, thyme, and garlic powder. Bring to a simmer over low heat and cook until thickened, whisking frequently to avoid clumps. This will take about 10 minutes.

4. Transfer broccoli to a cutting board and chop until it is the same size as the other vegetables. (If the florets are too large you will have trouble keeping your lasagna together). Place all roasted vegetables in a large bowl.

5. In a medium bowl, combine cottage cheese or ritocotta cheese, parmesan cheese, salt, pepper, garlic powder, oregano, and basil. Stir to combine.

6. Reduce oven temperature to 350 degrees and prepare your lasagna. Spray a 13 x 9 pan with nonstick cooking spray.

7. Spread about ½ cup of bechamel sauce on the bottom of the pan and place 3 lasagna noodles. Top with roasted vegetables, cheese mixture, a few handfuls of mozzarella cheese, and bechamel sauce. Continue with remaining layers until complete.

8. Bake for 45-50 minutes until bubbling. Allow to cool at least 45 minutes before slicing and serving.

Prep: 10 mins

Cook: 35 mins

Total: 45 mins

Servings: 4

Ingredients

- 4 bone-in, skin-on chicken thighs
- 1/3 cup honey
- 2 tablespoons balsamic vinegar
- 1 1/2 teaspoons dried Italian seasoning
- salt and pepper to taste
- 1 pound small red potatoes halved
- 1 tablespoon olive oil
- 1 pound asparagus stalks trimmed
- 2 tablespoons chopped parsley
- cooking spray

Directions

1. Preheat the oven to 425 degrees F. Line a sheet pan with foil, and coat the foil with cooking spray.

2. Arrange the chicken thighs on the pan. Season the chicken generously with salt and pepper.

3. In a small bowl whisk together the honey, balsamic vinegar and Italian seasoning.

4. Place the potatoes in a large bowl along with the olive oil, salt and pepper. Toss to coat.

5. Arrange the potatoes around the chicken. Brush half of the balsamic mixture over the chicken.

6. Bake for 20 minutes. Brush the remaining glaze over the chicken and add the asparagus to the pan. Season the asparagus with salt and pepper.

7. Bake for an additional 10-15 minutes or until chicken is done and potatoes and asparagus are tender.

8. Sprinkle with parsley, then serve.

9. Seared Scallops with Cheesy Acorn Squash Mash

Prep: 15 mins

Cook: 1 hr

Pureeing + Assembling: 15 mins

Total: 1 hr 30 mins

Servings: 4

Ingredients

Squash:

- 2 acorn squashes, halved
- 1 sweet potato
- Pure Avocado Oil
- Kosher salt
- 2 tablespoon unsalted butter cubed
- 2 garlic cloves minced
- 1/4 cup grated Emporium Selection Premium Aged Cheddar

Brown butter walnuts:

- 1/2 cup walnuts chopped
- 2 tablespoons unsalted butter
- Juice from 1/4 lemon
- 2 chives trimmed and minced
- Kosher salt
- Pinch of crushed red

Scallops:

- pepper
- 3 tbsp pure Avocado Oil
- 6 ounces frozen jumbo Scallops, thawed

Directions

To cook the squash:

1. Preheat your oven to 400 degrees F. Place acorn squashes on your baking sheet. Drizzle with a bit of oil and a few pinches of salt. Place face side down. Transfer to the oven to roast for 30 to 40 minutes, until tender.

2. Remove the squash from the oven and allow to cool for about 10 to 15 minutes, until they're cool enough to handle. Scoop the squash and add it to a food processor. Remove the skin from the sweet potato and add the sweet potato to the food processor, along with the butter, garlic, cheddar and a few pinches of salt. Process until mostly smooth. Give it a taste and adjust the salt according to taste.

To make the brown butter walnuts:

1. In a small pan, set over medium heat, add the walnuts and butter. Toast them until they're fragrant and slightly darker in color, about 2 minutes, until the butter is fragrant and turning a brown color. Mix in the lemon juice, chives, a pinch of salt and pepper. Set aside.

To cook the scallops:

1. In a skillet, set over medium high heat, add the avocado oil. When the oil is hot and glistening and glides along the pan smoothly. Add the scallops and don't move them until they begin to

lift off the pan, about 2 minutes. Flip the scallops and cook on their opposite side for 1 minute.

To assemble:

1. Add the squash to a platter and make a few swoops if you like. Top it with the scallops and spoon the brown butter walnuts on top. Serve immediately.

10. Chicken Enchiladas

Prep: 25 mins

Cook: 20 mins

Total: 45 mins

Servings: 6

Ingredients

- 2 tablespoons butter
- 1 medium onion chopped
- 2 tablespoons all-purpose flour
- 1 1/2 cups chicken broth
- 1 cup chopped green chile peppers
- 3 clove garlic finely chopped, more if desired
- 1 teaspoon Kosher salt or season to taste
- 1/2 teaspoon ground cumin more if desired
- 6 flour tortillas
- 1 cup shredded Monterey Jack cheese
- 1 cup shredded mild Cheddar cheese
- 2 cups shredded cooked chicken breast meat

- 1 cup heavy cream
- 1/2 - 1 cup any cheese to sprinkle over the top
- green onion & cilantro chopped for garnish

Directions

How to make Salsa Verde:

1. Using a pot, over medium heat, melt 2 tablespoons of butter then add 1 chopped onion, cook until soft about 3-5 minutes.
2. Stir in 2 tablespoons of all-purpose flour, cook for 1 minute, stirring continuously.
3. Pour in 1 1/2 cup of chicken broth. Then add 1 cup of chopped green chile peppers, 3 chopped garlic cloves, 1 teaspoon of Kosher salt and 1/2 teaspoon of ground cumin, simmer over medium/low heat for 5 minutes, stirring few times.

How to make Chicken Enchiladas:

1. Preheat your oven to 350F.
2. Dip 1 flour tortilla in the salsa Verde sauce, dip both sides. Put 1/4 cup of chicken breast in the

center of the tortilla. Sprinkle about 2 tablespoons of Monterey Jack cheese & 2 tablespoons of mild Cheddar cheese. Roll the tortilla into a roll, and place it in a baking dish.

3. Spread the rest of Salsa Verde sauce over the top of the enchiladas. Pour 1 cup of heavy whipping cream and sprinkle 1 cup of cheese. Place enchiladas in the oven & bake uncovered for 20 minutes.

4. Garnish with chopped green onion & cilantro. Serve with green lettuce & salsa.

11. Butternut Squash Mac and Cheese

Prep: 15 mins

Cook: 1 hr

Total: 1 hr 15 mins

Servings: 8

Ingredients

- Olive oil spray
- Kosher salt
- 1 pound cubed butternut squash
- 10 ounces whole wheat elbow pasta
- 1 ½ cups low sodium vegetable broth, divided
- ½ teaspoon onion powder
- ½ teaspoon garlic powder
- Freshly ground black pepper, to taste
- ¼ cup panko breadcrumbs
- 2 tablespoons freshly grated Parmesan cheese
- 1 tablespoon unsalted butter
- 1 medium shallot, minced
- ¼ cup all-purpose flour
- 2 cups skim milk

- ½ cup shredded gruyere cheese

- ½ cup shredded cheddar cheese

- Chopped chives, optional, for garnish

- Sriracha sauce, optional, for topping

Directions

1. Preheat oven to 375 degrees F. Spray a 9" x 11" glass baking dish with oil and set aside.

2. Bring a large pot of salted water to boil. Add squash and boil until tender, 5-6 minutes. When fork tender, transfer squash with a slotted spoon to a blender.

3. Add pasta to boiling water and cook according to package directions. When cooked, drain and put back into the pot.

4. Meanwhile, add ½ cup vegetable broth, onion powder, garlic powder, ½ teaspoon salt and pepper to the blender with the squash. Blend until smooth and creamy.

5. In a small bowl, combine breadcrumbs, Parmesan, ¼ teaspoon salt and pepper. Set aside.

6. Melt the butter in a medium sauce pot over medium heat. Add the shallots and sauté 2 minutes. Sprinkle the flour evenly over the shallots and cook for another minute.

7. Add the remaining 1 cup of broth and milk and whisk to combine. Bring sauce to a boil, then reduce heat to medium-low and cook for 5 minutes, whisking frequently.

8. Remove pot from heat and whisk in cheese, pureed squash, 1 teaspoon salt and pepper.

9. Add sauce to noodles, gently mix to combine, then transfer mixture to prepared baking dish.

10. Sprinkle with breadcrumb mixture and bake for 25 minutes. Switch oven to high broil and broil for 2-3 minutes, or until crumbs are starting to brown.

12. Summer Squash Pasta Skillet

Prep: 5 mins

Cook: 20 mins

Total: 25 mins

Servings: 4

Ingredients

- 8 ounces of your favorite pasta
- ¼ cup pine nuts
- 5 tablespoons unsalted butter
- 2 garlic cloves, minced
- 1 small zucchini squash, sliced into rounds
- 1 small summer squash, sliced into rounds
- kosher salt
- freshly cracked black pepper
- 4 ounces goat cheese, crumbled
- ¼ cup fresh basil leaves

Directions

1. Bring a pot of salted water to a boil and cook the pasta according to the directions.

2. While the pasta is cooking, heat a skillet over medium-low heat. Add the pine nuts. Toss and stir them until they are golden and fragrant, about 5 to 6 minutes. Remove from the heat immediately.

3. Heat a skillet over medium heat and add the butter. Whisk it constantly until brown bits begin to form on the bottom and the butter is golden. When that happens, add the garlic and squash rounds and toss to coat, then cook for 5 minutes until the zucchini softens. Sprinkle it with salt and pepper.

4. The pasta should be finished by now, so add it to the skillet with the zucchini. Turn the heat to low. Toss the pasta and squash well, making sure everything is combined and has a bit of butter on it. Crumble in the goat cheese and toss it well. Add in another few cracks of fresh black pepper. Toss in the pine nuts.

5. Stir in the fresh basil and serve immediately.

Prep: 10 mins

Cook: 50 mins

Total: 1 hr

Servings: 4

Ingredients

- 1 teaspoon olive oil
- 8 bone-in chicken thighs
- ½ teaspoon sea salt
- 4 red potatoes, chopped
- 1 head broccoli, chopped into florets
- Honey Mustard Sauce
- ¼ cup each: Dijon mustard and honey
- 2 tablespoons grainy mustard
- 1 large garlic clove, finely minced
- ¼ cup water

Directions

1. Preheat your oven to 400 degrees.

2. Heat the oil in a large, ovenproof skillet over medium-high heat. Add the chicken, skin-side up. Season the skin with sea salt. Cook the chicken for 5 minutes then flip it over and continue to cook it until the skin is brown, about 5 more minutes. While the chicken is cooking, chop the potatoes, 1 teaspoon olive oil,8 bone-in chicken thighs, and ½ teaspoon sea salt.

3. Remove the pan from the heat and place the chicken into a bowl. Add all the sauce ingredients to the pan and whisk them together. Add the potatoes and stir so they are coated in the sauce. Nestle the chicken between the potatoes and pour any accumulated juices (from the bowl the chicken was in) back into the pan.

4. Add ¼ cup each: Dijon mustard and honey,2 tablespoons grainy mustard,1 large garlic clove,¼ cup water, and 4 red potatoes.

5. Place the skillet in your oven and let it cook for 30 minutes. Carefully remove the pan from the oven and add the broccoli. Put the skillet back into the oven and cook for another 15-20 minutes, or until the potatoes are soft.

14. Peanut Sauce Chicken

Prep: 20 mins

Cook: 20 mins

Total: 40 mins

Servings: 6

Ingredients

- ½ cup natural, creamy peanut butter
- ½ cup hoisin sauce
- 2 tablespoons rice vinegar
- 1 tablespoons honey (or agave)
- 1 tablespoon chili garlic sauce (or your desired amount)
- 1 tablespoon soy sauce
- ½ cup water
- 1 ½ pounds skinless, boneless chicken thighs, cut into strips/chunks
- Salt
- Black pepper
- ¼ cup cornstarch

- Peanut oil (or your preferred variety good for high heat)
- 2 red bell peppers, cored and sliced into medium strips
- 6 cloves garlic, pressed through garlic press
- 1 teaspoon freshly grated ginger
- ½ cup peanuts, crushed or roughly chopped
- 2 green onions, sliced, for garnish
- 2 tablespoons cilantro leaves, for garnish

Directions

1. Prepare the peanut sauce by adding the peanut butter, hoisin sauce, rice vinegar, honey (or agave), chili garlic sauce, soy sauce and water to the bowl of a food processor, and process the ingredients until completely smooth and creamy; pour into a large cup or bowl, and set aside.
2. Add the chicken pieces into a bowl and season with salt and pepper, then toss to coat; sprinkle over the cornstarch, then toss once again to coat the chicken evenly.

3. Place a large heavy-bottom skillet over medium-high heat, and add in about ½ cup of the oil; once the oil is hot and shimmering, work in batches adding some of the coated chicken pieces to the pan, and allow them to sit, undisturbed, for about 3-4 minutes until a pale golden color and slightly crisp; stir to allow the chicken to brown on the other side for another minute or two, until cooked through; remove the chicken from pan and repeat with remaining chicken.

4. Next, turn the heat down under the pan to medium, and if needed, add a drizzle more oil; add in the red bell pepper strips, and quickly saute those until crisp yet still tender and vibrant, about 2 minutes.

5. Add in the garlic and the ginger, and stir to incorporate; once aromatic (about 30 seconds), add the chicken pieces back into the pan, stir to incorporate them with the peppers/garlic/ginger, then pour in the peanut sauce; stir to combine allowing the sauce to gently warm through for just a moment.

6. To finish the peanut sauce chicken, sprinkle in the peanuts and garnish with the green onions and cilantro leaves, and serve with rice or noodles.

15. Grilled Tahini Glazed Salmon with Cucumber
Noodles

Prep: 20 mins

Cook: 12 mins

Total: 32 mins

Servings: 2

Ingredients

- 1 pound salmon filet (about four 4 ounces portions)

Tahini Maple Sauce:

- 2 tablespoons tahini
- 2 tablespoons sesame oil
- 1 tablespoon sambal (garlic-chili sauce)
- 2 tablespoons maple syrup
- 1 tablespoon tamari (gluten free soy sauce or coconut amino acids)

For the Vinaigrette:

- ¼ cup rice wine vinegar

For The Noodles:

- 1 large English cucumber, turned into noodles
- 2 tablespoons toasted sesame sesame seeds

Directions

1. Preheat the grill to medium high.
2. On a sheet pan covered in foil, set the salmon filets directly on the foil.
3. In the jar of a blender, combine the ingredients for the Tahini Maple Glaze and puree on high until smooth.
4. Take 4 tablespoons of the tahini sauce and glaze the salmon with it.
5. Leave the remaining tahini sauce in the blender and add ¼ cup rice wine vinegar. Puree until smooth and then set aside.
6. Place the sheet of foil with the salmon filets directly onto the grill. Cook the salmon for 10-12 minutes or until the fish is just barely cooked through.

7. While the fish is cooking, in a large bowl, toss the cucumber with the vinaigrette (you may have extra dressing left over) and the sesame seeds.

8. Serve the grilled salmon on top of the dressed cucumber noodles.

16. Sesame Encrusted Chicken Tenders

Prep: 5 mins

Cook: 15 mins

Total: 20 mins

Servings: 4

Ingredients

- 8 chicken tenderloins, 18 oz total
- 3/4 tsp kosher salt and black pepper, to taste
- 2 tsp sesame oil
- 2 tsp low sodium soy sauce
- 6 tbsp toasted sesame seeds
- 1/2 tsp kosher salt
- 1/4 cup panko
- olive oil spray

Directions

1. Preheat oven to 425°F. Spray a baking sheet with non-stick oil spray.

2. Combine the sesame oil and soy sauce in a bowl, and the sesame seeds, salt and panko in another.

3. Place chicken in the bowl with the oil and soy sauce, then into the sesame seed mixture to coat well.

4. Place on the baking sheet; lightly spray the top of the chicken with oil spray and bake 8 to 10 minutes, until slightly browned on the bottom.

5. Turn over and cook another 4 - 5 minutes or until cooked through and the edges are crisp. Serve over rice with more soy sauce, if desired.

6. Preheat the air fryer. Cook for 10 to 12 minutes, flipping halfway until cooked through, crispy and golden.

17. Green goddess chicken salad phyllo cups
Prep: 15 mins

Total: 15 mins

Servings: 5

Ingredients

For the dressing:

- ½ of a ripe avocado
- ½ cup parsley
- ½ cup dill
- 2 cups baby spinach
- ½ cup Greek yogurt
- Juice of 1 lemon
- 2 tablespoons olive oil
- Salt and pepper, to taste

For the Phyllo Cups:

- ½ cup of the dressing (use as much as you like)
- 1½ cups cooked, diced chicken breast
- ½ cup halved red grapes

- ½ cup diced celery

- ¼ cup dried cranberries

- ¼ cup toasted sliced almonds

- 1 package frozen phyllo cups, defrosted

Directions

For the dressing:

1. Place all the ingredients in a food processor and pulse until everything is broken down and combined.

2. Scrape down the sides and run the machine a few more times to achieve a creamy, smooth consistency. Season, to taste, with salt and pepper.

3. Transfer the dressing to an airtight container and keep in the fridge for up to a week.

For the phyllo cups:

1. In a large bowl, combine the dressing, chicken, grapes, celery, half the cranberries, and half the almonds.

2. Spoon the mixture into the phyllo cups and garnish with the remaining cranberries and almonds. Serve chilled or at room temperature.

18. Parmesan Orzo with Mushrooms and Spinach

Prep: 10 mins

Cook: 20 mins

Total: 30 mins

Servings: 6

Ingredients

- 1 lb. orzo pasta

- 3 tbsp. olive oil

- 12 oz. mushrooms, chopped

- 10 oz. fresh spinach

- 1 tsp. garlic powder

- 1 tsp. onion powder

- 1 tsp. salt

- ½ tsp. freshly ground black pepper

- 2 tsp. oregano

- 1 cup parmesan cheese

- 4 tbsp. milk, cream, or half-and-half

Directions

1. Bring a large pot of salted water to a boil and cook orzo according to pasta directions. Drain and set aside.
2. Heat olive oil in the same pot. Add mushrooms and cook until tender, then add spinach and cook until wilted.
3. Return orzo to pot and stir to combine. Add garlic powder, onion powder, salt, pepper, oregano, and parmesan cheese and stir to combine.
4. Add milk, cream, or half-and-half and stir to combine. If you want more or less liquid in the pasta you can adjust to your taste.
5. Taste and adjust seasonings if needed.
6. Enjoy!

19. Mushroom Spinach White Pizza

Prep: 15 mins

Cook: 30 mins

Total: 45 mins

Servings: 2

Ingredients

- pizza dough of your choice
- 1 cup ricotta cheese, (plus 2-3 tablespoons, optional)
- ½ teaspoon salt
- ½ teaspoon Italian seasoning
- ½ teaspoon dried basil
- 1 package button mushroom, sliced
- 1 teaspoon butter
- ¼ teaspoon dried thyme
- 2-3 cups baby spinach leaves
- 1 teaspoon oil
- ½ teaspoon garlic powder

- ⅔ cup shredded mozzarella cheese

- Freshly ground black pepper

- ½ teaspoon red pepper flakes (optional)

Directions

1. Preheat the oven to 450 degrees Fahrenheit.

2. On a medium-size non-stick skillet, add the sliced mushroom and cook on high heat for a couple of minutes. The water from the mushroom will start to extract and evaporate.

3. Once the water from the mushroom started to evaporate and the mushroom turns slightly brown, add the butter and dried thyme to the mushroom. Stir frequently and cook for an additional minute or two. Take them off the skillet and set them aside.

4. On the same skillet, add the oil and spinach leaves. Sprinkle garlic powder and pinch of salt to the spinach and cook until all the spinach leaves are wilted, about 3-5 minutes.

5. When the spinach is wilted, take it off from the heat and set it aside.

6. In a small bowl, mix together 1 cup of ricotta cheese, ½ teaspoon of salt, ½ teaspoon of Italian seasoning, and ½ teaspoon of dried basil.

7. Divide the pizza dough in half.

8. Flour the working surface and start stretching the dough flat. Do the same for the other dough.

9. Spread the ricotta mixture to each of the stretched pizza dough evenly and thinly.

10. Add the cooked mushroom and spinach to both pizzas.

11. Add ⅓ cup of shredded mozzarella cheese (each) on top of the pizzas.

12. Sprinkle red pepper flakes if you like spicy pizza. If not, skip this step.

13. Sprinkle some freshly ground black pepper on top.

14. Place the pizzas in the oven and cook for 11-12 minutes.

15. Take them out of the oven and enjoy them right away.

20. Healing Morning Smoothie

Prep: 5 mins

Total: 5 mins

Servings: 1

Ingredients

- 1 cup coconut water
- 3/4 cup berries (or fruit of your choice)
- 1 tablespoon chia seeds (optional for extra protein)
- 1 tablespoon aloe vera
- 1/2 teaspoon probiotics
- 1/4 teaspoon coconut oil
- 1/4 teaspoon grated ginger

Directions

1. Blend everything in a high speed blender and drink right away.

21. Chicken Noodle Soup
Prep: 10 mins

Cook: 25 mins

Total: 35 mins

Servings: 4

Ingredients

- 1/2 tablespoon olive oil
- 1 cup celery, trimmed and chopped (about 2 stalks)
- 8 cups water
- 2 cups carrots, peeled and chopped (about 6 medium carrots)
- 4 low-sodium chicken bouillon cubes
- 1/2 teaspoon thyme
- 1/2 teaspoon salt
- 3 ounces dry large egg noodles
- 2 cups boneless and skinless chicken breasts, cooked and diced
- 2 cups frozen peas

Directions

1. Heat olive oil over medium-high heat in a large pot. Add chopped celery and cook until translucent.
2. Add water, carrots, chicken bouillon cubes, thyme, and salt to the pot. Bring to a boil.
3. Once boiling, add egg noodles to the pot and stir.
4. Reduce the heat to low and simmer. Cook for 8 minutes or until the noodles are tender.
5. Add the diced cooked chicken breast and frozen peas. Return to a boil.
6. Once boiling again, reduce the heat to medium-low. Cover and simmer for 5 to 10 minutes, or until the peas are warm and the soup has a flavorful aroma.
7. Serve the soup in individual bowls.

22. Chicken, Rice, & Vegetable soup

Prep: 15 mins

Cook: 30 mins

Total: 45 mins

Servings: 6

Ingredients

- 1–2 chicken breasts (11-12 oz total uncooked or 1 1/2 cups of cooked chicken)
- 1 cup of carrots, peeled and sliced (120 g)
- 1 cup of sliced celery (100 g)
- 1 cup of chopped asparagus (100 g)
- 1 cup of sliced white mushrooms (80 g)
- 4 cups of water
- 4 cups of chicken broth (or veggie broth)
- cooked jasmine rice
- 1 tbsp of olive oil
- 1 bay leaf
- 1–2 tbsp of fresh chopped parsley

- 1 tsp of sea salt or Himalayan salt

- pepper to taste (omit if not tolerated)

- Optional; fresh or dried thyme leaves and 1/8 tsp ground turmeric

Directions

1. Bring the water and broth to a boil in a stockpot. Then add the carrots, celery, chicken, bay leaf, and salt. Cover and simmer for 25-30 minutes (set a timer) or until chicken is cooked through.

2. While the soup is simmering, prepare the jasmine rice. Rinse your rice by pouring 1 cup of rice into a medium bowl. Fill the bowl with water until rice is completely covered. Stir the rice around using clean hands. Pour cloudy water out and repeat rinsing the rice a couple more times.

3. Add 2 cups of water to a saucepan and bring to a boil. Once boiling, add 1 cup of jasmine rice. Cover and reduce heat. Simmer for about 18 minutes-20 minutes without lifting the lid (time may vary depending on stove type). Fluff cooked rice with a fork and set aside.

4. 5 minutes before the timer for the soup goes off, add the asparagus to the stockpot.

5. Heat a skillet over medium heat, then add 1 tbsp of olive oil. Wait for the oil to heat up (1-2 minutes), then add mushrooms and a sprinkle of salt. Cook until tender (about 5 minutes), then add mushrooms to the stockpot.

6. Remove chicken from the stockpot and shred with a fork. Add the shredded chicken back to the soup.

7. Turn the heat off, remove the bay leaf from the soup, and add fresh chopped parsley, pepper, and more salt as needed. Add cooked jasmine rice to soup bowl after serving. Enjoy!

23. Carob Date Paleo Bread

Prep: 5 mins

Cook: 35 mins

Total: 40 mins

Servings: 16 thin slices

Ingredients

- 1 and 3/4 cup almond meal
- 1/4 cup ground flaxseed
- 1/4 cup coconut oil
- 1 tbsp coconut flour
- 1/4 cup carob powder
- 1 tbsp Date Syrup, just dates
- 1/2 tsp baking soda
- 1 tbsp Apple Cider Vinegar
- 1/8 tsp sea salt
- 5 eggs

Directions

1. Grease and flour a baking pan (you can use coconut flour).
2. Preheat oven to 350°F.
3. Combine almond meal, flaxseed, coconut flour, carob powder, coconut oil, date syrup, baking soda, apple cider vinegar and sea salt into a food processor and process until well combined.
4. Add eggs, one at a time, pulsing after each addition - until well blended.
5. Pour into prepared pan.
6. Bake for 25 minutes.
7. Cover with foil and bake another 10 minutes until firm, but moist.

24. Gluten-free Bircher Muesli

Prep: 15 mins

Soaking time: 6 hrs

Total: 6 hrs 15 mins

Servings: 5

Ingredients

- 275 g gluten-free rolled oats
- 80 g dried apricots, chopped
- 50 g pumpkin seeds
- 40 g almonds, roughly chopped
- 40 g pecans, roughly chopped
- 80 g ground almonds
- 30 g ground flaxseed
- 25 g hemp seeds
- 20 g sesame seeds
- 40 g homemade muesli - recipe above
- 80 g almond milk
- 60 g natural coconut yoghurt

- ½ apple, peeled and grated

- Handful of mixed berries

Directions

1. Mix all the ingredients together in a large mixing bowl.

2. Keep in a large storage jar until needed.

Bircher Muesli

1. Weigh out the muesli into an airtight container then stir in the milk, yoghurt and grated apple.

2. Place a tight fitting lid over the top then rest in the fridge overnight to soak.

3. Transfer the bircher muesli to a breakfast bowl, stir well then serve with the berries sprinkled over the top.

25. Acid Reflux Smoothie

Prep: 5 mins

Total: 5 mins

Servings: 1

Ingredients

- ¾ cup cashew milk
- 5 fresh basil (just leaves)
- ¼ cup spinach
- ½ inch ginger root
- 1 banana (frozen)
- ½ pear
- ⅓ cup rolled oats

Directions

1. Blend cashew milk, basil leaves, and spinach until smooth
2. Add remaining ingredients and blend again
3. Serve over ice for a refreshingly cool smoothie

26. Courgette Soup

Prep: 15 mins

Cook: 20 mins

Total: 35 mins

Servings: 2

Ingredients

- 1 Courgette (chopped)
- 1 Celery Stick (chopped)
- 1 tsp Olive Oil
- 400ml Vegetable Stock (make sure this is allergen free)
- 2 tbsp Chopped Almonds (toasted)
- Kale (2 big handfuls)
- 2 tbsp Fresh Basil (chopped)

Directions

1. In a clean pan toast the chopped almonds for a few minutes, being careful to not burn them, and carefully set aside.

2. In a large soup pan heat the olive oil on a medium heat. Add the chopped courgettes, celery and fresh basil and saute for 6 minutes.

3. Add the vegetable stock and bring to a boil. Reduce the heat to medium-low and then simmer for 10 minutes.

4. Add the two handfuls of Kale and simmer for another 5 minutes.

5. Stir in the toasted almonds and remove from the heat. Let it cool slightly.

6. In a blender, add the soup and puree in batches until smooth.

7. Add soup to the pan again and season with a good quality sea salt. Cook for a further 4 minutes on a medium to low heat.

8. Enjoy and serve with crusty bread if desired.

27. Cabbage Soup

Prep: 10 mins

Cook: 6 hrs 30 mins

Total: 6 hrs 40 mins

Servings: 2

Ingredients

- ½ green cabbage chopped
- 1 cup celery diced
- 1 cup onion diced
- 1 cup carrots sliced into thin coins
- 2 garlic cloves minced
- 4 cups vegetable broth (or chicken broth)
- 2 cups tomatoes diced
- 1 teaspoon oregano dry
- ½ teaspoon pink Himalayan salt
- ¼ teaspoon red pepper
- 2 tablespoons apple cider vinegar
- 1 teaspoon lemon juice

- 1 bay leaf dry

- 2 tablespoons gluten-free and vegan miso paste (or start with 1 tablespoon and add up to 3 tablespoons or to taste).

- 2 tablespoons parsley fresh, optional for garnish

Directions

Slow Cooker

1. In a slow cooker add all the ingredients. Cook for 4-6 hours on low. Serve right away garnished with fresh parsley.

Stovetop

1. Add all the ingredients in a large pot and turn the heat to medium high. When it starts to bubble on the sides, cover and turn the heat down to medium-low heat. Cook for about 20-30 minutes or until the carrots are soft.

28. Tomato-free pasta sauce

Prep: 10 mins

Cook: 30 mins

Total: 40 mins

Servings: 3

Ingredients

- 3 medium celery stalks
- 3 medium carrots, peeled
- 2 medium zucchinis
- 1 medium beet
- 1/2 a small-medium turnip, peeled
- 2 cups of bone or vegetable broth (or more as needed)
- 7–10 fresh basil leaves
- 3–4 tbsp of grapeseed oil or extra virgin olive oil
- 1 tsp each of garlic powder and onion powder (omit if unable to tolerate)
- 1/2 teaspoon of dried oregano

- 1 tsp of salt to add to sauce, plus a little more to season vegetables while cooking
- pepper to taste

Directions

1. Preheat oven to 400 degrees F.

2. Prep vegetables: Peel the carrots and turnip. Cut the leafy tops close to the top of the beet, and trim the ends off of the zucchini, celery, carrots and turnip. Cut vegetables (except beet) into two-inch chunks. Since we will only be using half of the turnip in this recipe, you can either cook all of the turnip or set the raw half that won't be used aside for use in other meals. Another option is doubling the recipe. Don't bother peeling the beet, as the skin is very tough to peel when raw. Peel it once it is cooked and slightly cooled.

3. Spread the cut up zucchini, carrots, celery, turnip and out onto a large rimmed baking sheet lined with parchment paper. Drizzle with 2-3 tbsps of grapeseed or olive oil and sprinkle with desired amount of salt and pepper, then cover using parchment paper, tucking it snugly underneath.

4. Wash the beet using a vegetable brush, then pat dry. Place in a baking dish lined with parchment paper and drizzle with 1 tbsp of olive oil. Cover using parchment paper, tucking the ends underneath.

5. Place vegetables in preheated oven and cook until they are tender and can be easily pierced with a fork. Stir the carrots, zucchini, celery, and turnip occasionally while cooking.

6. Once the beet is done cooking, let it cool slightly. Once cool, submerge it in a bowl of cold water and peel off the outer layer. Cut it in half and place that half in a high-speed blender or food processor. Feel free to add more if you want a deeper red color (keep in mind this will add a more earthy flavor to the sauce). Save the leftover beet for salads or other meals.

7. Add the remaining cooked vegetables, broth, and fresh basil to the blender. Process until you have a smooth consistency. Add the blended liquid to a saucepan along with the oregano, garlic powder, onion powder, salt, and pepper. Cook on medium-

low for 4-5 minutes while stirring. Add more broth as needed for a thinner consistency.

8. Remove from heat and serve with pasta or use as tomato/marinara sauce replacement.

29. Mediterranean Farro Salad with Arugula and Chickpeas

Prep: 10 mins

Total: 10 mins

Servings: 1

Ingredients

- 2 cups baby arugula
- 1/2 cup cooked farro
- 1 oz crumbled feta (about 1/4 cup)
- 1/3 cup garbanzo beans (chickpeas)
- 2 sweet cherry peppers
- a few splashes of balsamic vinegar
- 2 teaspoons olive oil
- fresh herbs, for garnish

Directions

1. Arrange ingredients into a large bowl or plate and drizzle with balsamic and olive oil. Sprinkle with a little salt and pepper to taste.

30. 10-minute Blackened Tilapia

Prep: 4 mins

Cook: 6 mins

Total: 10 mins

Servings: 2

Ingredients

Tilapia filets:

Vegetable Oil

Blackening powder recipe:

- 1 tbsp. smoked paprika
- 2 tsp. thyme
- 1 tsp. cumin
- 1 tsp. oregano
- 1 tsp. garlic powder
- 1 tsp. onion powder
- 1 tsp. salt
- 1/2 tsp. ground black pepper

- 1/2 tsp. ground red pepper

Directions

1. Mix dry ingredients together in a small bowl to create blackening powder. Then moisten the sides of each tilapia filet (either with water or cooking spray), and coat with blackening powder.
2. Heat 1 tbsp. of oil per filet in a skillet over medium-high heat. Once oil is almost smoking, add filets and cook for about 3 minutes per side, or until fish is opaque and can be flaked with a fork. Remove from pan and serve immediately.